A QUICK GUIDE TO

CBD

EVERYTHING YOU NEED TO KNOW

D1040347

A QUICK GUIDE TO
CBD

EVERYTHING YOU NEED TO KNOW

DR JULIE MOLTKE

An Hachette UK Company
www.hachette.co.uk

First published in Great Britain in 2020
by Gaia, an imprint of
Octopus Publishing Group Ltd
Carmelite House
50 Victoria Embankment
London EC4Y 0DZ
www.octopusbooks.co.uk
www.octopusbooksusa.com

Distributed in the US by
Hachette Book Group
1290 Avenue of the Americas
4th and 5th Floors
New York, NY 10104

Distributed in Canada by
Canadian Manda Group
664 Annette St.
Toronto, Ontario, Canada
M6S 2C8

ISBN 978-1-85675-437-8

A CIP catalogue record for this book is
available from the British Library.

Printed and bound in England

10 9 8 7 6 5 4 3 2 1

The information in this book is not
intended to replace or conflict with the
advice given to you by your doctor or
other health professionals. All matters
regarding your health should be
discussed with your doctor or other
health professional. The author and
publisher disclaim any liability directly
or indirectly from the use of the
material in this book by any person.

Commissioned by Emily Brickell
Senior Designer Jaz Bahra
Copy Editor Emma Bastow
Senior Production Controller
  Allison Gonsalves

CONTENTS

INTRODUCTION:
WHY LEARN ABOUT CBD

If you are reading this book it probably means that the hype around cannabidiol, or CBD for short, has not escaped your attention. And the hype is for good reason; the health and wellness community is honouring it for its anti-inflammatory and antioxidant properties, while celebrities have taken to social media to praise its role in managing stress and anxiety. Moreover, children with severe treatment-resistant epilepsy are experiencing an improvement in their symptoms when taking pure CBD medicine. Studies have shown that between 8 and 11 per cent of adults in the UK – approximately 4 to 6 million people – have tried CBD. In the US, 14 per cent of the adult population use CBD products, and among them 40 per cent use CBD for pain, 20 per cent for anxiety and 11 per cent to help them sleep. You may have considered it yourself, and it's no wonder when CBD is reported to help a wide range of conditions, from Post Traumatic Stress Disorder (PTSD) and insomnia to arthritis and menstrual cramps.

But how much do you actually know about this fascinating compound? You have probably realized that it comes from the cannabis plant and that it does not make you high, but did you know that CBD was discovered in 1942 by the American chemist Dr Roger Adams, who had a passion for plant chemistry? And did you know it has virtually no side-effects and no risk of addiction? Or that CBD can counteract the paranoid effects that cannabis (more specifically Tetrahydrocannabinol, or THC, see page 23) can have on the mind? You might have wondered what the best way to take CBD is or how it works in the body, and why it seems to have so many different effects. This simple guide, delivered to you by a doctor who has spent many years learning all there is to know about cannabis, will answer all of these questions and many more about one of the hottest topics of the decade.

CBD HEALTH AND SAFETY

Cannabis is generally thought to be safer than most drugs as it does not have a fatal toxic dose. THC can have some unwanted side-effects, but CBD is generally thought to be exceptionally well tolerated. A report by the World Health Organization states that CBD is considered a safe substance with little risk of abuse. A few pieces of advice for safe use:

- Always stick to the recommended dose.

- CBD may interact with other drugs such as blood-thinners and certain immunosuppressors. Always consult your doctor before taking CBD if you are taking other medications.

- Do not use CBD when pregnant or breastfeeding due to lack of evidence on the potential effects.

- Side-effects may include nausea, fatigue, light-headedness, irritability, change in appetite, low blood pressure and a dry mouth.

10,000 YEARS OF CANNABIS HISTORY

Before diving into contemporary uses of CBD, let's begin with a history of cannabis, the plant from which CBD is derived. Humans have had a relationship with cannabis for thousands of years; it is thought to be one of the earliest plants used for medicinal purposes. It is only in the past 100 years or so that cannabis has been subject to prohibition.

Cannabis is indigenous to the steppes of central China and the Indian subcontinent, where it was traditionally used in the manufacture of fibre and textiles, as well as as a medicine and for religious ceremonies. The first recorded medical use of cannabis, for pain relief and anaesthesia, dates to about 4000 BCE. According to an ancient Chinese myth Shen Nung, the Red Emperor, used the cannabis plant for agriculture and medicine around 2700 BCE. He is believed to have written the *Shen Nung*

Pen Ts'ao (The Herbal), which is still in use by practitioners of Traditional Chinese Medicine today, and includes more than 300 medicines derived from plants, animals and minerals.

However, as historians cannot confirm the existence of the Red Emperor, whether he was a myth or a real figure will probably remain a mystery.

Even though exact figures and dates are unconfirmed, there is little doubt that the cannabis plant was widely used in central Asia, and seeds have been found in graves in Siberia and northern China dating back more than 4,000 years. Humans and cannabis have had a friendly co-existence for more than 10,000 years; it is only during the past century that it has been perceived as a threat to society and our health and wellbeing.

> **Humans and cannabis have had a friendly co-existence for more than 10,000 years; it is only during the past century that it has been perceived as a threat.**

On the Indian subcontinent hemp was known by the Sanskrit name *ganja,* and cannabis appears under the name *soma* in *The Vedas,* one of the oldest and most holy Indian texts, dating back to 2000 BCE. Cannabis is used by Ayurvedic practitioners today and was traditionally used for its psychoactive properties in religious rituals and for its known effects to treat conditions such as grief, gout and aches and pains. The word *bhanga*, closely related to the modern word *bhang*, meaning edible cannabis, also appears in several ancient Indian texts.

From central Asia the cannabis plant travelled from India and China to the Middle East and Europe with nomads who used it as a 'camp flower' – a plant they took with them when they moved. When the Spanish set out to discover the New World they brought cannabis with them, and from there it spread to South and North America. The list of uses in ancient civilizations ranges from easing symptoms of epilepsy, neuralgia and anxiety, to managing chronic pain, tumours and migraine. The effect of cannabis on many of these conditions is being investigated by modern researchers.

It is interesting to consider that the continent where cannabis was last introduced, but first prohibited, is the place it is now most widely used for medicinal, wellness and recreational purposes.

RECENT HISTORY

Cannabis was widely used as a medicine all over the world during the 19th century and could be found in various preparations in pharmacies. William O'Shaughnessy, an Irish doctor, is famous for having introduced cannabis to western medicine when returning from India in 1841. He had experimented with cannabis

CHARLOTTE'S STORY

CBD took its most significant leap into the hall of fame in 2013 with the release of the movie *Weed*, a documentary by the American neurosurgeon Dr Sanjay Gupta. *Weed* follows the captivating story of Charlotte, a little girl with Dravet syndrome, a severe form of treatment-resistant epilepsy. Charlotte was having more than 300 seizures a week and did not respond to traditional treatment. She was introduced to the Colorado-based Stanley Brothers who had developed a high CBD cannabis strain, later named Charlotte's Web after the little girl. The world was touched by how cannabis transformed the life of Charlotte and her family when she became almost seizure-free when using CBD oil.

Similarly, medicinal cannabis was legalized in the UK in November 2018 following the campaigning by the parents of Billy Caldwell and Alfie Deacon, two boys with severe treatment-resistant epilepsy, who were forced to illegally import cannabis or move country to make sure their children had access to the medicine they needed.

on his patients and had found that it could relieve the spasms caused by tetanus infection in infants, as well as pain from rheumatism. Over the following decades, cannabis was often used to treat various ailments. However, with the introduction of pain-relieving medicines such as morphine and aspirin, based on single molecules, cannabis was forgotten by the medical profession. At the same time an opium epidemic was sweeping the world and cannabis was dragged into the war on drugs, hence since 1925 it has been an internationally controlled drug.

In recent years both CBD and cannabis have relaunched into the health and wellness world, primarily from the legalization of recreational and medicinal cannabis in several states in the US and Canada, followed by many countries in Europe. Though there is still controversy around the legality of CBD, it is now used and loved by millions of people across the world for its

Despite the efforts to prohibit CBD, it is slowly but surely making its way back into our medicine cupboards.

anti-anxiety, anti-inflammatory, antioxidant, anti-seizure, anti-spasmodic, pain-relieving, anti-depressant and anti-nausea effects. Despite the efforts to prohibit CBD, it is slowly but surely making its way back into our medicine cupboards and taking up its rightful place as a safe and natural medicine.

CBD SCIENCE
FOR BEGINNERS

To kick off our science class, let's start with the basics: where does CBD come from? CBD is an organic chemical compound from the cannabis plant. Traditionally three species have been recognized within this category: *Cannabis sativa*, *Cannabis indica* and *Cannabis ruderalis*, although some researchers and taxonomists have argued that it is likely they are all subspecies of *Cannabis sativa*.

This seems simple, but let's go a little further. Under the above categories there are more than 800 different cannabis strains, and numbers are increasing as different hybrids emerge all over the world. These strains have been cultivated to have different chemical profiles, so-called chemotypes or chemovars, often classified by their content of CBD and THC (see page 25).

ONE PLANT WITH MANY EFFECTS

A chemovar is the specific chemical footprint of a plant within a certain plant family (genus). Just like identical twins might look the same while having completely different personalities, different cannabis strains might look pretty similar but have different cannabinoid, terpene and flavonoid (see page 27) profiles, and exert different effects when used by humans. The 800 plus different strains can have slight differences in their chemovar and thereby be used for different medical and recreational purposes. The cannabis plant contains more than 500 different chemical compounds, although not all of these contribute to the unique properties of the plant.

THE HEMP VS MARIJUANA STORY

One of the most confusing things for a newcomer in the cannabis world can be the nomenclature used to describe the plant. CBD comes from hemp; hemp comes from cannabis and is legal in most countries, whereas marijuana, which also comes from cannabis, is illegal in most countries. If this does not make any sense to you, you are not alone. Although hemp and marijuana both belong to the same species of cannabis, *Cannabis sativa*, the difference between them for legal purposes is the content of THC. Hemp contains less than 0.2–0.3 per cent THC while marijuana can contain up to 40 per cent THC.

Hemp is a strain of *Cannabis sativa* that is grown for industrial purposes to yield a vast amount of fibre while producing minimal amounts of THC. Hemp is not usually traded as an illegal drug as it is unlikely to make anyone high, which is the purpose of most illicit drugs. Hemp plants, on the other hand, can be used to make CBD.

CBD can also be made from other cannabis strains with a higher percentage of THC. The THC can then be removed from the extract to meet the legal

CBD comes from hemp; hemp comes from cannabis and is legal in most countries, whereas marijuana, which also comes from cannabis, is illegal in most countries. If this does not make any sense to you, you are not alone.

requirement of the country where it is sold. For example, at the time of writing, in the UK there should be no traces of THC in the CBD sold in stores, even though it is legal to grow hemp with up to 0.2 per cent THC. In the US, the law differs from state to state; some states have legalized recreational or medical cannabis while others still prohibit it. CBD derived from hemp with less than 0.3 per cent THC is, however, legal in all states in America.

These legal terms and nomenclature can be confusing even for the people in the CBD industry. A market analysis of 30 CBD products available in stores in the UK found that 45 per cent of the products contained small traces of THC. Although not enough to get you high, this means they were basically illegal.

MEET THE CANNABINOIDS

The phytocannabinoids ('phyto' meaning from a plant) are a family of chemical compounds found in abundance in the cannabis plant. They are also found in small amounts in other plants such as echinacea, often used to prevent or treat the common cold. Before attacking that old bottle in your bathroom cupboard, remember that these compounds won't get you high as they do not contain any THC.

There are more than 100 different cannabinoids known to date. While this book focuses on CBD, to fully understand this compound we need to meet the family, beginning with tetrahydrocannabinol, the famous big brother of CBD.

A TALE OF THC

Tetrahydrocannabinol, or THC, is the most prominent and highly famed cannabinoid in the cannabis plant, renowned for its intoxicating effect. THC was responsible for the 1970 classification of cannabis among the Class 1 Schedule of drugs, which also includes cocaine and heroin, making it almost impossible to conduct clinical research (Class 1 substances are drugs with no accepted medical use and at high risk of abuse). THC binds directly to the cannabinoid receptor (see page 32) in the brain and by activating it can lead to well-known side-effects, including increased appetite, changes in perception and mood, a dry mouth and occasionally feelings of anxiety or paranoia.

These are familiar effects for anyone who has tried recreational marijuana. But for the medicinal cannabis user, most of these symptoms would indicate that you have used too much and are considered side-effects. THC, when used for medicinal purposes (as opposed to recreational use), is known to relieve chronic pain, especially neuropathic pain arising from a damaged or inflamed nervous system. It can help with sleep issues, decrease vomiting and nausea and relax muscles. It is also known to have anti-inflammatory and antioxidant properties, which can explain the effects seen in people with irritable bowel syndrome (IBS) and other diseases with an element of chronic inflammation. In my experience patients who use medicinal cannabis containing THC often experience a decrease in perceived pain levels, improved sleep and an increased quality of life.

THE RISING STAR OF THE CANNABINOIDS

Cannabidiol, better known as CBD. If the cannabinoids are a boy band, CBD is Robbie Williams: the lucky favourite who ran away for a solo career and earned all of the fame. CBD was discovered decades before THC, but for a long time it seemed like a one-hit-wonder, without the star status that it has today. Throughout the history of cannabis cultivation, the aim has always been to grow strains with a chemical profile with as much THC and as little CBD as possible.

Cannabidiol, better known as CBD. If the cannabinoids are a boy band, CBD is Robbie Williams: the lucky favourite who ran away for a solo career and earned all of the fame.

CBD differs from THC in many ways, but the most important difference is the way it works in the brain. CBD is non-intoxicating and does not have the potential to make you high like THC. A common misunderstanding is that CBD is not psychoactive. This is not entirely true; CBD works on receptors in the brain and is therefore by definition psychoactive (see page 58).

CBD is the second most prominent cannabinoid in cannabis after THC, and it can be sold as a food supplement without a prescription in many countries. CBD is loved for its anti-anxiety, anti-depressant and anti-seizure effects. Studies have shown that it has anti-inflammatory and antioxidant properties, and that it can protect neurons, also called nerve cells. Studies even showed CBD to have anti-bacterial effects (see page 56) and that it can help wound healing. And if all that isn't enough, you can add pain relief and muscle relaxation to the list.

The story of Charlotte (see page 14) and other children around the world who have seen an improvement in their treatment-resistant epilepsy with the use of high CBD strains, and research into the many beneficial properties of CBD, have placed CBD in the spotlight where it belongs.

THE PARENTS, AUNTS AND UNCLES

THC and CBD might be the most famous and prominent cannabinoids in the clan, but the family includes more than 100 members. None of these have been explored to the same degree as THC and CBD, but they also have distinct personalities and unique qualities that can help to treat a variety of conditions. Without getting caught up in a long conversation with the crazy uncle, let me introduce you to a few other cannabinoids.

The mother of all cannabinoids is cannabigerolic acid (CBGA), and she is transformed into both THC and CBD with a little help from enzymes in the trichomes (a part of the cannabis flower). CBGA is non-intoxicating and studies show that it can protect nerve cells as well as being a potent anti-inflammatory and antioxidant agent.

THC and CBD might be the most famous and prominent cannabinoids in the clan, but the family includes more than 100 members.

Both cannabidiolic acid (CBDA) and tetrahydro-cannabinolic acid (THCA) are found in raw, unheated cannabis flowers; when heated they are transformed to CBD or THC. This is what happens when lighting a joint or when the dried cannabis flower is vaporized. They do however have properties in their own right, and some people make extracts from the dried flowers to benefit from this.

Cannabinol (CBN) is found in ageing cannabis and is created by the oxidation of THC. It has anti-bacterial and anti-inflammatory properties, among others.

Lastly there's tetrahydrocannabivarin (THCV), which blocks the cannabinoid receptor, thereby suppressing appetite and giving high hopes for a new anti-obesity agent.

TERPENES AND FLAVONOIDS

The terpenes and flavonoids can be seen as the younger cousins of THC and CBD. If you like to use broad- or full-spectrum oils these will be part of the mix and this explains why some people prefer these oils over oils made from CBD isolates (see page 63). They are not cannabinoids but still have their claim to fame, and they are receiving a growing level of well-deserved attention due to their many benefits in the human organism. Terpenes are essential oils and can be found in most plants, adding to their distinct smell.

There are around 200 terpenes found in cannabis and they vary from strain to strain, which explains why some strains have different effects even though they have the same content of THC and CBD. Some important terpenes include:

Limonene
Potent anti-depressant and anti-anxiety effects. Also found in citrus rind and peppermint. Enhances the anti-depressant and anti-anxiety effects of CBD.

Linalool
Anti-anxiety, analgesic, sedating and calming effects. Also found in lavender and coriander.

Beta-myrcene
Sedating, muscle relaxing and analgesic. Most common terpene in cannabis and responsible for the distinct smell. Not found in hemp.

Beta-caryophyllene
Anti-inflammatory and analgesic effects, gastrointestinal relief and protection. Also found in black pepper, cloves and hops.

Approximately 20 flavonoids are found in cannabis, and they are responsible for the plants' pigmentation. Studies have shown that flavonoids can have antioxidant and anti-inflammatory effects and are able to combat fungus, bacteria and viruses.

Flavonoids are thought to protect against certain kinds of cancers. The three most prominent flavonoids in the cannabis plant are Cannaflavin A, Apigenin and Quercetin.

THE ENTOURAGE EFFECT

You have now learned the basic facts about the cannabis plant and the colourful family of organic compounds found within it. However (without sounding too clichéd), as the writer Ryūnosuke Satoro once said, 'Individually, we are one drop. Together, we are an ocean.'

This also seems to be the case for the cannabinoid, terpene and flavonoid families. When all the different compounds in the cannabis plant are used together (as whole plant extracts) they seem to exert synergism, meaning that together they have an effect that is greater than the sum of their isolated properties. This is known as the entourage effect. CBD and THC have been shown to increase the effect on pain when used together, and while CBD alone might not help you sleep, the right combination of cannabinoids and terpenes in a certain strain can help to induce a peaceful slumber.

The entourage effect has not yet been scientifically proven but the empirical and clinical data strongly supports this idea, as do many of the researchers and clinicians at the forefront of the cannabis industry.

THE AMAZING ENDOCANNABINOID SYSTEM

It may seem as though you cannot open a wellness magazine without reading about CBD, or pick up a newspaper without noticing an article on medicinal cannabis. Politicians talk about it, millions of people use it and yet doctors knowingly ignore it. Despite this interest, not many people are talking about the answer to most cannabis-related questions: the endocannabinoid system (ECS). The ECS is a large part of the reason why CBD and cannabis have so many different effects and why people use it to treat everything from anxiety to menstrual cramps. Read on to find out more...

RECEPTORS, SYNAPSES AND MESSENGERS

If you were the kind of kid who sat in the last row in biology class doodling and looking out of the window, you need not worry – we will stick to the basics and keep it short. The ECS is a biological system involved in maintaining the balance of an organism, or homeostasis in geek language (see page 83). It consists of three elements:

The receptors

Receptors are turned on and off to regulate processes in the body. The receptors are sitting on our nerve cells, and they can be compared to a docking station in a harbour. When the dock is empty there is not much activity, but when ships are docking the whole environment of the harbour changes. The receptors of the endocannabinoid system are called cannabinoid receptors. The most well-known are the CB1 and CB2 receptors, but there are more than 20 known receptors in the ECS to date.

THE NEUROTRANSMITTERS

The messenger molecules in the endocannabinoid system are called endocannabinoids, and they are produced in our nerve cells in response to a disturbance in our internal environment. The endocannabinoids bind to the docking station like ships, to balance the activity between cells in our body. There are many different endocannabinoids; the most studied are called Anandamide (from *ananda*, the Sanskrit word for bliss) and 2-Arachidonoylglycerol (2-AG).

The enzymes
The enzymes are like the people unloading the ship so it can leave the harbour. The enzymes are responsible for breaking down the endocannabinoids and thereby returning the receptors to their resting state, reintroducing peace in the harbour.

When an endocannabinoid binds to the cannabinoid receptor and activates it, the main effect is to 'turn down the volume' – the ECS gets feedback from messengers within the body when some signals have become too loud. By activating the CB1 and CB2 receptors, they help turn down the signal volume and keep the environment comfortable and tidy.

You now know about the main parts of the ECS and how they are involved in balancing your physiological and mental processes in response to changes in your external environment. However, this is an oversimplified picture. The complexity of this system is hard to grasp, even for the most dedicated researchers, and we will probably see that there is still more to discover about the ECS in the future.

THE OMNIPRESENT ENDOCANNABINOID SYSTEM

The ECS is a bit like social media; it reaches everywhere and controls everything. This may be an exaggeration, but as you learn more about the endocannabinoid system and what it does you will understand.

The ECS has receptors in the central nervous system (including everything inside the brain and the spinal cord), the peripheral nervous system and immune cells. There are more cannabinoid receptors in the brain than anywhere else in the body and they by far exceed the number of opioid receptors (the receptors that both endorphins and morphine bind to), which have effects on pain, feeling of euphoria and physical dependence.

The brain primarily has CB1 receptors (see page 32), and they are positioned in abundance in areas that are involved with the sensation of pain, memory and learning, emotion, motor control and appetite. Receptors are also found in areas of the brain associated with nausea and vomiting, which explains why CBD and THC can ease these symptoms. One of the greatest things about CB1 receptors is that they are not present in the area of the brain involved with the breathing control: the brain stem. This is the reason why a cannabis overdose isn't fatal, as opposed to an overdose of drugs like morphine, fentanyl

THE WOMAN WHO NEVER FEELS PAIN AND IS ALWAYS HAPPY

Jo Cameron, a 66-year-old Scottish woman, amazed doctors when she did not need standard pain treatment following surgery for severe arthritis. Tests revealed that she had two gene mutations that caused a decrease in the activity of FAAH, the enzyme that breaks down the endocannabinoid anandamide. Doctors then discovered that her circulating levels of anandamide in the blood were twice as high as usual. Anandamide is involved in mood, memory and pain sensation. When asked, it turned out that Jo had always felt extraordinarily happy, never felt stressed or anxious, and she did not feel pain like normal people. The latter had resulted in a lot of burns, bruises and broken bones, and probably also led to the severe arthritis that resulted in the operation in the first place. Jo told the doctors that she had always been very forgetful, and she never bore a grudge. All these traits seemed to be linked to her high levels of anandamide.

and oxycodone. Every medical professional knows that even over-the-counter medicines such as paracetamol can kill or cause irreversible liver damage when taken in excess.

Outside of the brain, CB1 receptors are found in the lungs, vascular system, liver, heart, pancreas, reproductive organs, skin and muscles. CB2 receptors are primarily found on various immune cells and help to regulate inflammation and balance the immune system. The peripheral nervous system also has CB2 receptors, as does the brain, bone tissue, heart, liver, gastrointestinal tract, reproductive system and the skin. So some tissues express only CB1 or CB2 receptors, while others express a combination of both.

The most important take-away is how widely the ECS is spread across the body; this is why cannabinoids have so many different effects.

THE IMPORTANCE OF THE ENDOCANNABINOID SYSTEM

The ECS is involved in controlling mood, memory, fear, sleep, anxiety and stress levels. It also regulates pain, gut health, immune function, hunger, fertility and reproduction, blood sugar levels and metabolism and bone growth.

The ECS is like the head butler in a grand hotel. You hardly notice him, but he makes sure the guests are comfortable, the hotel is always the perfect temperature, the rooms are clean, the pillows are soft and the flowers are fresh. As with the butler, you often don't notice when the ECS is working and things are flowing as they should. But when there is an imbalance in the system it is likely to manifest as physical or emotional symptoms, and then all hell breaks loose.

The endocannabinoid system is like the head butler in a grand hotel. You hardly notice him, but he makes sure the guests are comfortable, the hotel is the perfect temperature, the rooms are clean, the pillows are soft and the flowers are fresh.

The American neurologist Ethan Russo, who is one of the most influential researchers and clinicians in the cannabis world, has suggested that many common diseases result from an imbalance in the ECS. In 2003 he hypothesized that low levels of endocannabinoids in the body could lead to common conditions such as migraines, fibromyalgia and IBS. Unexplained physical symptoms such as these have caused doctors headaches for decades, and in desperation some have been characterized as somatoform, or functional disorders: a smart way of saying 'we have no clue why people get this, and it might all be in your head'. Needless to say there are not many good treatment options for people with these kinds of conditions, which has left millions of doctors and patients across the globe in frustration. Luckily, research is helping us move away from these stigmatizing classifications.

It has long been known that disturbances in our neurotransmitter levels can cause diseases. A lack of serotonin is associated with depression and other mental illnesses, while a dopamine deficiency is associated with Parkinson's disease. It should therefore be no surprise that disturbances in the ECS can also cause havoc in the body and lead to clinical conditions with no other obvious cause. Later research has supported Ethan Russo's idea, and the list of conditions with a proposed element of endocannabinoid deficiency has now grown to include Huntington's disease, anxiety, depression, multiple sclerosis, Parkinson's and other common treatment-resistant conditions.

CAN I CONTROL MY ENDOCANNABINOID SYSTEM?

You might ask what this means for you on a day-to-day basis. Can you actually control your ECS? It has been shown that by changing your diet and decreasing stress levels, you can upregulate the function of the ECS. In my experience as a doctor, many chronic diseases can be reversed by changing to a healthier lifestyle. The key elements should be an anti-inflammatory diet, reducing daily stress levels by approved methods such as mindfulness, meditation, yoga or other exercises, and last and most importantly getting enough sleep (7–9 hours). CBD can also help to balance the ECS and treat many of the conditions mentioned further on in this book (see pages 46–56).

CBD AND THE ENDOCANNABINOID SYSTEM

CBD is not the kind of cannabinoid to cut corners and has many roles to play in the body. CBD interacts with the ECS in several different ways, as well as working with other essential systems in the body. Surprisingly to many, and as opposed to THC, CBD cannot activate the cannabinoid receptors (see page 32). Even though it does not have the ability to bind directly to the docking site, it can still interact with the CB1 receptor in a way that blocks the binding of other molecules to the receptor. Returning to the harbour analogy, we can think of CBD as sailing around in front of the harbour without docking, and thereby blocking the way for other ships to reach the dock. This is the reason why CBD can weaken the effects of THC and decrease the paranoia often associated with marijuana use.

CBD HAS A GOOD INFLUENCE ON THC

When CBD interacts with the CB1 receptor in the presence of THC, it can attenuate many of the effects of THC. For users of medicinal cannabis, a balanced ratio of CBD to THC can be valuable. Too much THC can cause fear and paranoia, and the high can be accompanied by feelings of losing control. However, when balanced with CBD there is a good chance that medicinal cannabis will not make you high, paranoid or anxious.

You might be wondering, therefore, if CBD counteracts all of the effects of THC. Is that what we want, after hearing how THC can alleviate chronic pain, nausea, vomiting and other common symptoms? The answer is no, CBD does not attenuate all the effects of THC. Studies have shown that our two favourite cannabinoids work synergistically (creating an effect that is greater than the mere sum of the two parts). THC and CBD together can often treat chronic pain symptoms more effectively than if used alone.

CBD AND THE HORMONE OF BLISS

CBD has been shown to increase levels of the endocannabinoid anandamide by inhibiting FAAH, the enzyme that breaks down this blissful neurotransmitter. Remember the example of Jo Cameron, who was always happy-go-lucky, never felt depressed or stressed out and hardly felt any pain (see page 35)? It is this increase in anandamide that is responsible for many of CBD's positive effects.

CBD'S SIDE-JOBS

We now know that CBD does not directly activate the CB1 and CB2 receptors, but instead interacts with the system in more subtle ways. We know that CBD can counteract some of the effects of THC, while also working synergistically to enhance other effects. But some of the most-loved properties of CBD are not explained by its interaction with the ECS.

CBD binds to and activates the 5HT1a receptor. This seems to be the key to decreased anxiety levels, and the anti-depressant and the anti-psychotic effects people observe when using CBD. CBD also binds to another very interesting receptor called PPAR-γ. Research shows that this might help people suffering from movement disorders such as Parkinson's and Huntington's disease. CBD interacts with many other targets in the body not mentioned here. However I did promise you that I wouldn't go into so much detail that you're left looking empty-minded out of the window, so I shall move on to the next section of the book, the clinical effects of CBD.

A SMALL NOTE ON CANNABIS AND PSYCHOSIS

The link between cannabis and psychosis has undoubtedly been one of the biggest arguments against the use of medicinal cannabis. It is worth mentioning that this risk seems to be connected to smoking illegally obtained, and therefore unregulated, cannabis with THC levels up to 30–40 per cent (known as 'skunk'). Medicinal cannabis does not contain these high percentages of THC, and the CBD is a protective factor. At Clinic Horsted, a pain clinic in Denmark, we have treated more than 4,000 patients with medicinal cannabis and not one has experienced even a single episode of psychosis.

THE MANY BENEFITS OF CBD

We have learned about the origins of cannabis, where CBD comes from, how it is made and how it works in the body. We now have all the background information needed to move on to what might be the most exciting part of the book – what CBD does. First, a small warning.

A LACK OF CLINICAL EVIDENCE

Before we learn about the properties of CBD, it is essential to look at the latest research. Even though CBD has been studied for many decades, clinical trials to support the observed effects are still lacking, with the exception of epilepsy (see page 49). We have piles of studies looking at the effects of CBD in animals such as mice, and we have endless case reports and observational data. Still, at the time of writing, we do not have many big studies looking at the effects of CBD on humans. In the medical world, to really prove that something works it isn't enough that a lot of people use it and say that it works for them. Well-designed studies of a certain group size are needed, where one half of the group receives the drug (CBD), and the other receives a placebo (a pure oil without any cannabinoids). The participants in the clinical trial would be randomized to receive either the drug or a placebo, and neither the participant nor the researcher would know who received what. These are called randomized, double-blind, placebo-controlled trials (RCT) and are considered the gold standard.

You might think that it is crazy we cannot use observational data to determine whether something works or not. However, RCTs are there to make sure that a drug is effective, safe and not just a placebo. The placebo effect is when a person experiences an improvement when given a placebo substance without any active ingredients. This effect is attributed to the person's belief that the treatment is working.

In the following pages, I will explore the potential effect of CBD on conditions that it has been found to help.

CBD AND... AUTISM AND ADD/ADHD

Children with autism often experience symptoms such as aggression, hyperactivity and anxiety that can be difficult to manage. Dr Bonnie Goldstein, one of the most experienced and dedicated paediatricians, has been using cannabinoids to help treat children with severe autism and ADD/ADHD (Attention Deficit Disorder/Attention Deficit Hyperactivity Disorder) in her medical centre in California with excellent results for years. In Israel, where the use of medicinal cannabis and cannabis research is more advanced than anywhere in the world, studies have supported the use of CBD in treating symptoms of autism and ADHD.

How to use
Always consult your doctor before giving CBD to children, no matter what the clinical indication, and follow their advice.

CBD AND... CANCER

Patients with cancer often find that cannabinoids can help relieve the accompanying symptoms of pain, nausea and vomiting, loss of appetite and anxiety. Many people find that by improving sleep, general mood and quality of life, medicinal cannabis helps them get through their cancer treatment. Some individuals have claimed that they have a CBD oil to treat cancer. This is a dangerous and false claim which might make people abandon their conventional treatment and trade it for cannabis oil with no evidence but anecdotal case reports. Until we have the results of human trials, we simply cannot say whether cannabis can treat certain forms of cancer or not. What we do know is that both THC and CBD have anti-cancer properties for certain kinds of cancer. Pre-clinical research shows that CBD can induce cell death in certain types of breast cancer and gastric cancer, and can reduce tumour size in certain lung cancers. Animal trials also show that CBD has anti-tumour effects on a specific type of brain tumour called glioma.

How to use
Always talk to your doctor before using CBD if you have a been diagnosed with cancer as CBD might interfere with certain chemotherapies. CBD can, however, be a great help for people coping with the disease by decreasing the stress and anxiety associated with having cancer.

CBD AND... EPILEPSY

Treatment-resistant epilepsy accounts for approximately 30 per cent of the total number of epilepsy cases and is associated with serious outcomes for the patients. Children who suffer from this kind of epilepsy usually end up far behind their peers, have severe intellectual disabilities and mortality rates are high. Parents of sufferers are often desperate as they see their children having up to several hundred seizures per day. Several gold-standard RCTs have shown that CBD can help reduce seizures in children with Dravet syndrome and Lennox-Gastaut syndrome, and decrease the frequency of the seizures by almost 50 per cent. Many clinicians report patients who became almost seizure-free when using CBD, or a high CBD:THC ratio. At the time of writing, CBD under the name of Epidiolex is approved by both the American FDA (Federal Drug Administration) and the NHS (National Health Service) in the UK, although the fact remains that not many doctors prescribe it.

How to use
CBD for epilepsy is an oral solution which is used sublingually if possible. Always consult with your doctor before taking CBD for epilepsy.

CBD AND... INFLAMMATION

CBD has many desirable properties that are highly sought after in our modern wellness society. First, it is an antioxidant, which means it can protect our cells from toxic damage. Second, it is neuroprotective, meaning it can protect our nerve cells from damage (see page 84). Third and most importantly, it is a potent anti-inflammatory agent.

The anti-inflammatory properties are thought to be one reason why CBD might be useful in treating many chronic diseases with elements of chronic inflammation. These include many forms of arthritis, diabetes and gastrointestinal inflammatory illnesses such as ulcerative colitis and Crohn's disease (two chronic and often invalidating inflammatory bowel diseases). CBD might also be useful to treat the pain and inflammation associated with chronic hepatitis C infection.

How to use
CBD can be taken as a daily supplement as part of your anti-inflammatory regime. 50–70mg sublingual CBD oil (see page 65), potentially combined with a CBD cream, should do the trick.

CBD AND... MENTAL HEALTH

One of the most promising territories for CBD is mental health. With conditions such as stress, anxiety and depression increasing across the world, people are looking for natural remedies and CBD is among the front runners. Several studies show that the ECS is altered in people with depression, and this was also seen in examined brains of depressed people who committed suicide.

In a small clinical trial, participants with social phobia were given a high dose of CBD or a placebo before performing in a public speaking test. The result showed that CBD could decrease associated anxiety. CBD is also known to help reduce symptoms of PTSD and schizophrenia, and it might have a role to play in combating addiction and managing the opioid epidemic that claims hundreds of lives across the world every day.

Lastly, CBD may help prevent the progression of Alzheimer's disease, characterized by inflammation and the formation of beta-amyloid plaques in the brain followed by dementia.

How to use

If you tend to have minor depressive episodes, such as during winter when there is less daylight, try taking CBD once or twice per day, adjusting the dose until you feel an effect. Use a CBD oil with a terpene profile high in limonene (see page 27), which has an anti-depressant effect.

CBD AND... MOVEMENT DISORDERS

Both Parkinson's and Huntington's disease are movement disorders associated with neurodegeneration and damage to the nerve cells in some regions of the brain. There are promising results for the use of cannabinoids to treat the symptoms associated with Parkinson's, such as tremors, rigidity and cognitive symptoms including depression and anxiety. As we have seen CBD can protect nerve cells, and it may even have a role to play in preventing the progression of these diseases.

The ECS also seems to be involved in Tourette syndrome, a neurological disorder with involuntary repetitive movements and verbal tics, and cannabinoids seems to be able to reduce these symptoms.

How to use
Many Parkinson's patients report that adding a daily dose of CBD oil to their treatment regime greatly helped reduce the severity of their symptoms.

CBD AND... PAIN

Pain can be divided into two categories, acute and chronic, where the latter is pain that lasts for longer than 12 weeks. Cannabis is not particularly effective against acute pain as the ECS does not have a big role in the regulation of the processes involved. Other systems such as the opioid system are working when it comes to acute pain, and this is why morphine and its derivatives work much better than cannabis. It is a different story altogether when it comes to chronic pain. To put it simply, chronic pain can be divided into nociceptive pain, also called musculoskeletal pain, arising from joints or muscles, and neuropathic pain, resulting from damage to the central or peripheral nervous system, or a combination of both.

There is good evidence to support that cannabis is a well-tolerated treatment for chronic pain in around half of the patient population. It is especially useful for treating neuropathic pain like fibromyalgia (a condition characterized by chronic diffuse pain all over the body, sleep disturbances, IBS and fatigue), nerve damage or pain associated with tumours or spinal cord injury. As well as reducing chronic pain, cannabis is also known to improve sleep and general quality of life. Sativex, a sublingual spray containing THC and CBD in the ratio 1:1, is approved as a treatment for pain and muscle stiffness in multiple sclerosis patients.

How to use

CBD can work wonders for chronic pain, however many people with chronic pain will not experience adequate pain relief by using CBD alone. In my experience of working with CBD, it is most effective in conditions such as arthritis, migraine, chronic headaches and fibromyalgia, among others. Any chronic pain with an element of inflammation is also likely to benefit from CBD.

CBD AND... THE SKIN

We have an abundance of CB1 and CB2 receptors in the skin, and the endocannabinoid system seems to be involved in both cell growth and wound healing. Many of the most common skin conditions, including psoriasis, acne and allergic contact dermatitis, are characterized by inflammation of the skin. CBD has been shown to reduce inflammation and sebum secretion in people with acne, reduce inflammation associated with contact dermatitis as well as inhibit the growth of tumour cells in skin cancer patients.

How to use
You can use a CBD-containing cream to help reduce skin redness or to treat mild acne. Apply at night as part of your evening skincare routine.

CBD AND... SLEEP

Sleep is one of the most important factors for maintaining good mental health. Among CBD users, it is the third most popular reason to use CBD, after pain management and anxiety. Many people report sleeping better when using CBD, and I often hear from users that it becomes easier for them to switch off. Users also tend to feel less anxious, which makes it easier to fall asleep. We do, however, still need human clinical trials to truly know how CBD affects sleep patterns.

How to use
Try taking CBD in an evening blend containing other sleep-promoting ingredients, such as roman chamomile or valerian root. Oils or capsules, taken 1–2 hours before bedtime, can help a busy mind to wind down.

CBD AS AN ANTI-BACTERIAL AGENT

Studies show that CBD can kill certain bacteria when applied to a growth medium and researchers are looking at the possibilities of using it to combat bacterial infections. We need promising new treatments like this to help reduce the massive use of antibiotics, which is leading to a rise in multi-resistant bacteria with fatal consequences.

COMMON MISUNDERSTANDINGS ABOUT CBD

As with all celebrities, CBD is often misunderstood and misinterpreted. Here we will explore some of the biggest misunderstandings people often have about CBD. After finishing this book, you will be a promising CBD expert and able to entertain around the dinner table with some of these CBD facts.

CBD IS NOT PSYCHOACTIVE

This is one of the biggest misunderstandings in cannabis literature. CBD *is* psychoactive as it interacts with receptors in the brain and regulates our mental processes in subtle ways. This is the reason why it works for conditions such as anxiety and stress. What people mean when they say CBD isn't psychoactive is that it is not psychomimetic (mimicking symptoms of psychosis) and cannot make you high.

CBD WAS RECENTLY DISCOVERED

We have known about CBD for decades. It was first isolated from the cannabis plant in the early 1940s by the American chemist Dr Roger Adams. Nearly 20 years later the molecular structure was determined by Dr Raphael Mechoulam, the godfather of cannabis research.

CBD ONLY COMES FROM THE HEMP PLANT

CBD can be isolated from hemp plants, but it is also found in marijuana plants (see page 19). In fact, hemp and marijuana are the same plants, only the amount of THC, the intoxicating cannabinoid, differs. European hemp typically contains less than 0.2 per cent THC.

CBD IS FOR STONERS

This idea could not be further from the truth as CBD does not make you high. CBD is for everyone; from stressed-out bankers to grandmothers with arthritis and earth mothers with anti-inflammatory nutrition plans and yoga mats under their arms.

CBD IS A WONDER DRUG

CBD is not a panacea. It can't stop you from experiencing worrying thoughts or take away chronic pain. What it can do is help alleviate many physical and mental symptoms when used as a tool alongside a healthy lifestyle and other holistic modalities. CBD is not a substitute for traditional pharmaceuticals, but can be used alongside conventional western medicine.

A CBD USER'S GUIDE

You have now gathered enough knowledge about CBD to dive into one of the most confusing areas of the CBD hype: how to use it. In this section we will go over all you need to know, from choosing a product to deciding on dose and delivery method.

CBD products are most commonly made from hemp or cannabis strains with a high CBD content. The CBD is dissolved in a carrier oil such as MCT (medium-chain triglycerides) or hemp oil – CBD is naturally fat-soluble, but certain technologies exist to make CBD water-soluble.

CBD PRODUCTS ARE BROKEN DOWN INTO THREE CATEGORIES

ISOLATES: Pure 99.9 per cent CBD with terpenes, flavonoids and other cannabinoids removed.

BROAD-SPECTRUM: Contain CBD and the other components of the cannabis plant including terpenes and the minor cannabinoids CBG and CBN (see page 26). The THC has been removed.

FULL-SPECTRUM: Similar to broad-spectrum but also containing THC.

Since THC is an illegal substance in most countries, full-spectrum products are usually not available to purchase. Some people believe that broad-spectrum products are more beneficial than isolates because of the entourage effect (see page 29) created when terpenes and cannabinoids work together. However, there is not currently enough research to determine this sufficiently.

CBD DELIVERY METHODS

Capsules and tablets

Humans don't like change. For a new trend to really catch on, the user needs to recognize it and feel comfortable using it. CBD capsules, tablets and soft gels have been very successful in the CBD marketplace, probably due to their familiar form and ease of use – they are easy to take and look a lot like other health supplements. The downside is that they might not deliver the most value for money as only a small amount of CBD reaches the bloodstream. As with most drugs taken orally, CBD undergoes a 'first pass metabolism' in the liver and digestive tract before reaching the bloodstream. When taken orally it can take up to two hours before the effects of CBD are felt, and the effects usually last for 6–8 hours. Capsules and tablets are typically available in strengths from 5mg to 25mg.

Edibles

There is a vast list of CBD edibles available, catering to all requirements, including mints, gummies, chocolates, coffees and even lagers. Edibles are a great way to take CBD discreetly or more casually, and are excellent as top-ups throughout the day. Similar to capsules and tablets, the amount of CBD reaching the bloodstream may be limited due to the 'first pass effect' (see above) in the liver and digestive tract.

Oils and tinctures

Probably the most popular way of using CBD, sublingual products are a great choice as they avoid the 'first pass effect' (see opposite). CBD is absorbed underneath the tongue, bypassing the digestive tract and thus becoming available more quickly and effectively. Oils and tinctures are also a good option if you would prefer to avoid sugar and preservatives, which are common components of edibles.

Oils and tinctures make it easier to alter or fine-tune your dose than capsules with a fixed dose. Taken under the tongue and left there for as long as possible, at least 1–2 minutes, the solution is absorbed by the superficial blood vessels at the bottom of the mouth. If you stick out your tongue and lift it, you can see the blood vessels under the delicate mucous lining of the mouth. Tinctures and oils usually come in similar bottles but are slightly different: oils contain CBD mixed in a carrier oil, whereas tinctures are usually CBD dissolved in alcohol, which can conceal the strong taste of CBD.

Topicals

Topical creams, balms and sprays are useful for treating localized conditions and are a good option if you don't feel comfortable with the systemic effects (the effects on the whole body) of CBD. Topicals can be great at treating skin issues such as itches, wounds, eczema and acne. When choosing topical products check the product description for mentions of nano-technology, encapsulation or micellization – this ensures the CBD will penetrate through the dermal layers of your skin rather than remaining on the surface.

Transdermal

Unlike topicals, the drugs contained in skin patches cross the dermal barrier to enter the bloodstream. They release small amounts of CBD, usually over 4–6 hours, which is activated by body heat. Matrix patches are infused with a CBD in the adhesive layer. Reservoir patches have a small reservoir of CBD combined with a gel solution and are thought to offer a more controlled and steadier delivery system than matrix patches.

Vaporizing

Vaping has become increasingly popular over the past decade. CBD can be vaped either as an e-liquid or as the dried CBD flower. When using a vape, the CBD is heated to 200°C (392°F) and inhaled as a vapour. This is probably the quickest method of getting CBD into the bloodstream as it is absorbed through the small blood vessels in the lungs. However, it is also effective for the shortest amount of time and requires more continual usage. As vaping is a relatively new phenomenon, we do not yet have the research needed to evaluate the health effects of vaping

CBD. Be sure to purchase e-liquid only from licensed producers and retailers and be aware that you should never use alcohol-containing tinctures for vaping due to their high flammability.

Other ways to use CBD

CBD is being used in all kinds of places: in the bedroom, while relaxing in the bathtub and even on tampons. As well as in the forms covered in the last few pages, CBD can also be found in products ranging from personal lubricants and arousal sprays to bath bombs, pillow mists, body scrubs, suppositories and scented candles. Although the hard science backing these products is still limited, their use can probably add to a general feeling of relaxation, which many of us long for after a stressful day.

USING CBD FOR THE FIRST TIME

Many people will have a certain amount of anticipation when trying CBD for the first time. Whether or not they have used recreational cannabis, the possibility that they might feel high is often in the back of their minds. Regardless of the expectation most people are surprised, or even a little disappointed, when they try CBD for the first time as nothing much seems to happen.

Depending on how CBD is taken, the effects can be compared to a regular painkiller; you don't feel anything when taking it but soon after, the pain eases. CBD works in subtle ways that can be hard to detect directly, but the effects help the organism to adapt and stay balanced.

Before using CBD for the first time, it can be a good idea to do a bit of research. Reading this book is a great way to quickly become a CBD connoisseur, but the internet is also full of articles with tips and tricks. Before you get started you might want to ask yourself the questions below.

THREE QUESTIONS TO ASK YOURSELF BEFORE TAKING CBD

1. Why do you want to try CBD?

2. Which effects are you looking for?

3. Do you have a preferred application method (oil, topical, capsules)?

A SAMPLE USER

You suffer from mild social anxiety and have tried therapy with some effect but are still bothered by attacks from time to time. You want something to take the edge off when your anxiety is at its worst and have heard that CBD might help. Your commute to work is a trigger, as is being in the office when the atmosphere is too hectic. You investigate the different ways of taking CBD and find out that vaping gives the fastest result. Trying it, you feel calmer already after a few minutes. But you quickly realize that you need something longer lasting. After speaking to the manager at the local CBD store, you try a medium-strength CBD oil and take 25mg in the morning and after lunch. You now only need the vape on rare occasions, which is excellent as you never really like the feeling of vaping.

FINDING THE RIGHT PRODUCT FOR YOU

Finding the product that works for you can be tricky, and you might have to go through a bit of trial and error before discovering the right brand and delivery method. If you have a general inflammatory pain condition such as IBS or fibromyalgia, you will be best off using oil or capsules. If you have trouble with anxiety and stress, oils or vape might be able to help you out. Some people use CBD as a general supplement for its anti-inflammatory, antioxidant and neuroprotective properties, and again, for this purpose, oils or capsules can be of great use.

Testing whether you prefer to use an oil from CBD isolate or a broad-spectrum oil can also be a good idea. Some oils have added terpenes with unique properties, and your product search can be further refined by selecting specific terpenes. If you are having trouble sleeping, you might want to try a product with the terpene beta-myrcene, while anxious people can benefit from a CBD oil with added linalool. Producers have also added other beneficial ingredients like chamomile or ashwagandha to enhance and refine the effects of the CBD.

GET THE DOSE RIGHT

Let's get down to the practicalities of using CBD. You've done your research, and you are about to purchase your first product. You've decided to use an oil, ordered it online from a trusted source and now it's time to try it for the first time. Oils usually come in 10ml or 30ml bottles and a standard pipette can contain 1ml or 20 drops, but this may vary. Let's make it easy and say you bought a 10ml bottle containing 1000mg of CBD. You now know that 1ml contains 100mg, and 1 drop contains 5mg. One general piece of advice is to start low and go slow, increasing the dose every 3–5 days until you can feel the desired effects.

SAMPLE DOSES

1. **Days 1–5:** 3 drops (or 15mg) under the tongue for 2 minutes in the morning

2. **Days 5–10:** 3 drops morning and evening (30mg daily dose)

3. **Days 10–15:** 6 drops morning, 3 drops in the evening (45mg daily dose)

4. **Days 15+:** 6 drops morning and evening (60mg daily dose)

This is just an example, and your dose needs to be adapted to your individual needs. My endocannabinoid system is not the same as your endocannabinoid system, which is not the same as your friend's, so this really is all about personal fine-tuning which can take time, patience and money.

In accordance with the guidelines at time of writing, I do not recommend taking more than 70mg per day without consulting a doctor. CBD at the doses recommended above are considered extremely safe and with very few side-effects.

WHAT TO LOOK FOR IN A CBD PRODUCT

The CBD market is highly unregulated and random tests have found that only a few of the products on sale contain what it stated on the bottle. So, the very first thing to look for when choosing a CBD product is quality control. Any CBD brand or retailer should be able to show a certificate of control from a third-party lab stating what is in the product. This should state the cannabinoid and terpene content, and show that it does not contain any solvents, heavy metals or pesticides. As the industry is shaping itself, several regulatory bodies are appearing. This allows smaller brands to sign up to umbrella organizations that have testing facilities and offer advice to their members. In the long run, brands that do not take these things seriously will not survive. Furthermore, brands that are not serious about quality control are risking the future of the industry. For the CBD industry to survive, even the smallest brands must follow standard procedures that guarantee users a safe product, containing exactly what is says on the bottle.

The Association for the Cannabinoid Industry (ACI) is one such regulatory organization, helping its members to maintain high quality control. On their website (www.theaci.co.uk) you can find the brands that follow the guidelines in their CBD charter.

SAFETY MEASURES AND DRUG INTERACTIONS

CBD in doses of up to 1000mg daily has been taken safely for many weeks at a time without serious side-effects. However, until we have more extensive clinical trials to establish the safety profile and effective dose fully and in accordance with the guidelines at time of writing, I recommend not taking more than 70mg per day. If you need to go higher than this, it might be time to speak to your doctor.

FIVE CBD RULES

1. Do not take CBD when pregnant or breastfeeding.

2. Always talk to your doctor if you are considering taking CBD alongside other medications to make sure there are no severe interactions.

3. Speak to your doctor before starting using CBD if you are suffering from a cardiovascular disease.

4. If you are taking CBD in addition to cancer treatment or immune-therapy, always let your doctor know.

5. Don't give CBD to children except on the recommendation of a doctor.

Due to lack of evidence, it is safest to abstain from using CBD during pregnancy and breastfeeding unless advised by your doctor. CBD is metabolized by a group of liver enzymes called Cytochrome P450. Several other drugs, including certain blood-thinners, are metabolized by the same CYP450 enzymes. Therefore CBD might alter the activity of these drugs. At the clinic I work at in Denmark we have treated thousands of people with medicinal cannabis without seeing any such interactions, but if you are unsure whether CBD might interact with your current medication, always consult your doctor.

THE FUTURE OF CBD

As a simple medical doctor, it is hard to foresee the future of CBD. Fortune tellers and financial experts might be able to give a better view. However, as a rising star it seems that CBD is set to claim an important place in both the wellness and medical worlds. In the wellness industry, where products are not necessarily backed by decades of research, CBD is already acknowledged for its anti-inflammatory and antioxidant properties, and is used after exercise and as an integrated part of a healthy lifestyle.

Whether CBD will remain available as a food supplement in stores is entirely down to the regulatory bodies in various countries. At the time of writing, CBD is considered a novel food in Europe (a food that does not have a significant history of consumption). Brands that intend to import or manufacture CBD-containing foods into this area are therefore required to submit a CBD novel food application before sale. The regulation will likely change in the coming years, and this will determine how easy it will be to access CBD products. Another question is the price; as the scale of production increases the prices will drop, and hopefully we will see a range of more affordable CBD products coming onto the market.

I think that in the next decade we will see cannabis slowly moving away from the prison of prohibition to find a place in the daylight.

It is likely and much needed that CBD's role in the medical world will be defined in the years to come. The many clinical indications where CBD might be beneficial need to be determined and clarity needs to be sought on whether CBD is a medicine, a food supplement or both. I think that in the next decade we will see cannabis slowly moving away from the prison of prohibition to find a place in the daylight. Cannabis is not a wonder drug, but it can be part of the solution to many of the medical and existential problems faced by humanity today.

KEY TERMINOLOGY

ACTIVITY

Cannabinoid A class of diverse chemical compounds that acts on cannabinoid receptors in cells that alter neurotransmitter release in the brain.

Phytocannabinoid Cannabinoids that occur naturally in the cannabis plant, including THC and CBD.

Endocannabinoid Endogenous (occurring naturally in the body) neurotransmitters that bind to cannabinoid receptors (e.g. Anandamide and 2-AG).

Receptor An organ or cell able to respond to external stimulus and transmit a signal to a sensory nerve (e.g. CB1 and CB2).

Ligand A molecule that binds to a target protein, such as a receptor, and has the power to modulate a receptor's behaviour. Cannabinoids are ligands; they bind to CB1 and CB2 receptors.

Endocannabinoid system (ECS) A system of endocannabinoids and receptors in the body's central and peripheral nervous system, playing an important role in regulating and mediating a variety of physiological and cognitive processes, including homeostasis.

Homeostasis The stable state of an organism and of its internal environment; the equilibrium of all the body's functions.

Entourage effect A concept and proposed mechanism by which cannabinoids have a stronger impact together than as individual cannabinoids taken separately.

QUALITIES AND BENEFITS

Anti-inflammatory Refers to the property of a substance or treatment that reduces inflammation or swelling.

Anticonvulsant Agents used in the treatment of epileptic seizures.

Antioxidant A molecule that inhibits the oxidation of other molecules. Oxidation is a chemical reaction that can produce free radicals, leading to chain reactions that may damage cells.

Antiemetic Effective against vomiting and nausea.

Anxiolytic Medication or other intervention that inhibits anxiety.

Antipsychotic A class of medication primarily used to manage psychosis (including delusions, hallucinations, paranoia or disordered thought), principally in schizophrenia and bipolar disorder.

Analgesic Pain relieving.

Antispasmodic Used to relieve involuntary muscle spasms.

Anti-tremor A chemical agent that reduces unintentional, rhythmic muscle movement, involving oscillations of one or more parts of the body.

Immunomodulatory A chemical agent that modifies the immune response or the functioning of the immune system.

Neuroprotective May result in salvage, recovery or regeneration of the nervous system, its cells, structure and function.

SCIENTIFIC RESEARCH

Clinical trial Experiments and observations in a clinical research environment.

Randomized trial A type of scientific experiment, often in the medical field, where the people being studied are randomly allocated one of the different treatments.

Anecdotal report A description of the medical and treatment history of one or more patients from personal accounts, observations or the analysis of individual clinical cases, rather than the study of scientifically randomized groups of patients.

Placebo A substance with no active therapeutic effect, such as a sugar pill or injection of sterile water, given under the guise of effective treatment.

Placebo effect The total of all non-specific effects, both good and adverse, produced by a placebo drug or treatment, which cannot be attributed to the properties of the placebo itself, and must therefore be due to the patient's belief in that treatment.

RESOURCES

This is a selection of references used in writing this book. For more information and further references, please contact the publisher or writer.

1. Pertwee, R. (2016). *Handbook of Cannabis*. Oxford: Oxford University Press.
2. Goldstein B. (2016). *Cannabis Revealed: how the world's most misunderstood plant is healing everything from chronic pain to epilepsy.*
3. Mücke, M., Phillips, T., Radbruch, L., Petzke, F. and Häuser, W. (2018). Cannabis-based medicines for chronic neuropathic pain in adults. *Cochrane Database of Systematic Reviews*.
4. Whiting, P., Wolff, R., Deshpande, S., Di Nisio, M., Duffy, S., Hernandez, A., Keurentjes, J., Lang, S., Misso, K., Ryder, S., Schmidlkofer, S., Westwood, M. and Kleijnen, J. (2015). Cannabinoids for Medical Use. JAMA, 313(24), p.2456. Available from: http://www.ncbi.nlm.nih.gov/pubmed/26103030
5. Babson, K., Sottile, J. and Morabito, D. (2017). Cannabis,

Cannabinoids, and Sleep: a Review of the Literature. *Current Psychiatry Reports*, 19(4). Available from: http://www.ncbi.nlm.nih.gov/pubmed/28349316

6. Nielsen, S., Germanos, R., Weier, M., Pollard, J., Degenhardt, L., Hall, W., Buckley, N. and Farrell, M. (2018). The Use of Cannabis and Cannabinoids in Treating Symptoms of Multiple Sclerosis: A Systematic Review of Reviews. *Current Neurology and Neuroscience Reports*, 18(2).

7. Lal, S., Prasad, N., Ryan, M., Tangri, S., Silverberg, M., Gordon, A. and Steinhart, H. (2011). Cannabis use amongst patients with inflammatory bowel disease. *European Journal of Gastroenterology & Hepatology*, 23(10), pp.891–896. Available from: http://www.ncbi.nlm.nih.gov/pubmed/21795981

8. Bergamaschi, M., Queiroz, R., Chagas, M., de Oliveira, D., De Martinis, B., Kapczinski, F., Quevedo, J., Roesler, R., Schröder, N., Nardi, A., Martín-Santos, R., Hallak, J., Zuardi, A. and Crippa, J. (2011). Cannabidiol Reduces the Anxiety Induced by Simulated Public Speaking in Treatment-Naïve Social Phobia Patients. *Neuropsychopharmacology*, 36(6), pp.1219–1226. Available from: http://www.nature.com/articles/npp20116

9. Crippa J., Zuardi A., Hallak J. (2010). Therapeutical use of the cannabinoids in psychiatry. *Brazilian Journal of Psychiatry*, 32 Suppl 1:S56–66.

10. Devinsky, O., Patel, A., Cross, J., Villanueva, V., Wirrell, E., Privitera, M., Greenwood, S., Roberts, C., Checketts, D., VanLandingham, K. and Zuberi, S. (2018). Effect of Cannabidiol on Drop Seizures in the Lennox–Gastaut Syndrome. *New England Journal of Medicine*, 378(20), pp.1888–1897. Available from: http://www.ncbi.nlm.nih.gov/pubmed/29768152

11. Tóth, K., Ádám, D., Bíró, T. and Oláh, A. (2019). Cannabinoid Signaling in the Skin: Therapeutic Potential of the "C(ut)annabinoid" System. *Molecules*, 24(5), p.918.

12. Russo, E. (2011). Taming THC: potential cannabis synergy and phytocannabinoid-terpenoid entourage effects. *British Journal of Pharmacology*, 163(7), pp.1344–1364.

13. Di Marzo, V. (2008). The endocannabinoid system in obesity and type 2 diabetes. *Diabetologia*, 51(8), pp.1356–1367.

14. Ehrenkranz, J. and Levine, M. (2019). Bones and Joints: The Effects of Cannabinoids on the Skeleton. *The Journal of Clinical Endocrinology & Metabolism*, 104(10), pp.4683–4694.

15. Russo, E. (2016). Clinical Endocannabinoid Deficiency Reconsidered: Current Research Supports the Theory in Migraine, Fibromyalgia, Irritable Bowel, and Other Treatment-Resistant Syndromes. *Cannabis and Cannabinoid Research*, 1(1), pp.154–165.

16. McPartland, J., Guy, G. and Di Marzo, V. (2014). Care and

Feeding of the Endocannabinoid System: A Systematic Review of Potential Clinical Interventions that Upregulate the Endocannabinoid System. *PLoS ONE*, 9(3), p.e89566.

17. National Academies of Sciences, Engineering, and Medicine (2017). *The Health Effects of Cannabis and Cannabinoids*. Washington, D.C.: National Academies Press. Available from: https://www.nap.edu/catalog/24625

18. Hindocha, C., Cousijn, J., Rall, M. and Bloomfield, M. (2019). The Effectiveness of Cannabinoids in the Treatment of Posttraumatic Stress Disorder (PTSD): A Systematic Review. *Journal of Dual Diagnosis*, 16(1), pp.120–139.

19. Zuardi, A., Crippa, J., Hallak, J., Moreira, F. and Guimarães, F. (2006). Cannabidiol, a Cannabis sativa constituent, as an antipsychotic drug. *Brazilian Journal of Medical and Biological Research*, 39(4), pp.421–429.

20. Müller-Vahl, K. (2013). Treatment of Tourette Syndrome with Cannabinoids. *Behavioural Neurology*, 27(1), pp.119–124.

21. Kleckner, A., Kleckner, I., Kamen, C., Tejani, M., Janelsins, M., Morrow, G. and Peppone, L. (2019). Opportunities for cannabis in supportive care in cancer. *Therapeutic Advances in Medical Oncology*, 11, p.175883591986636. Available from: https://www.ncbi.nlm.nih.gov/pubmed/31413731

22. Health Canada. (2018). *Information for Health Care Professionals: cannabis (marihuana, marijuana) and the cannabinoids*. Canada: Health Canada

INDEX

ACKNOWLEDGEMENTS

My first book is dedicated to my friends and family who have supported me on my journey to where I am today.

Pushed by a feeling of never fitting into the established Danish medical system, I took the first baby steps into the wilderness of paths unknown to me and ended up as a holistic cannabis doctor in London. There is freedom and empowerment in such a journey but also fear and sometimes a lack of belief in oneself; at these times you were always there for me.

Walking down this road has led me to fight for a more holistic approach in western medicine; to push for a shift from symptom treatment to a time of prevention and lifestyle medicine. I want to thank my partner for his patience and calm as I rush around the world trying to build what I believe in.

I also want to thank my mentors and my colleagues who have supported me and believed in me, you all know who you are.

Lastly, I want to dedicate this book to everyone who is on the brink of taking that leap of faith into following their passion; remember, all big journeys start with a small step in the right direction.